Understanding

CHILDREN'S
EAR, NOSE & THROAT ILLNESSES

Dr D.P. Addy

GW00481790

Published by Family Doctor Publications Limited
in association with the British Medical Association

IMPORTANT NOTICE

This book is not designed as a substitute for personal medical advice but as a supplement to that advice for the patient who wishes to understand more about his/her condition.

Before taking any form of treatment YOU SHOULD ALWAYS CONSULT YOUR MEDICAL PRACTITIONER

In particular (without limit) you should note that advances in medical science occur rapidly and some of the information contained in this booklet about drugs and treatment may very soon be out of date.

© Family Doctor Publications 1996
Reprinted 1998

Family Doctor Publications, 10 Butchers Row, Banbury, Oxon OX16 8JH

Medical Editor: Dr Tony Smith
Consultant Editor: Chris McLaughlin
Cover Artist: Dave Eastbury
Medical Artist: Angela Christie
Design: MPG Design, Blandford Forum, Dorset
Printing: Reflex Litho, Thetford, using acid-free paper

ISBN: 1 898205 21 3

Contents

Introduction

Ear, nose and throat problems are among the most common childhood ailments, causing a great deal of upset to your child and worry to you as parents. This booklet aims to explain these problems so that you understand them better. It is meant to be used in conjunction with consultations with your GP, but not as a substitute for them. It can be difficult to decide exactly what is wrong with a child – especially a very young one – and usually a doctor is the only person

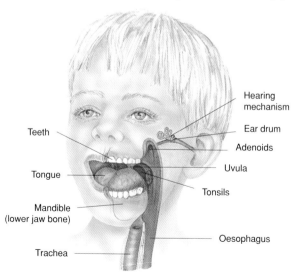

Teeth

Tongue

Mandible
(lower jaw bone)

Trachea

Hearing
mechanism

Ear drum

Adenoids

Uvula

Tonsils

Oesophagus

The main structures in the nose and throat

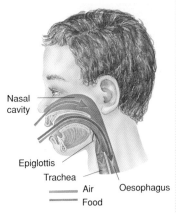

Nasal cavity
Epiglottis
Trachea
Oesophagus
=== Air
=== Food

The pathways taken by food and air after they enter the mouth and nose

who can make an accurate diagnosis. Illness does not affect just one part of the body in isolation – there is inevitably a considerable overlap with problems affecting other nearby parts. The ears, nose and throat are no exception and some of the disorders discussed here originate in nearby areas such as the chest. On average, young children have around six 'colds' each year so it's hardly surprising that they also succumb frequently to secondary illnesses such as ear infections.

This will be easier to understand if we first look at the diagram of the head and neck on page 1 showing where the various body parts we'll be discussing lie in relation to one another.

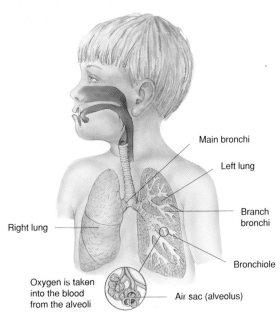

Main bronchi
Left lung
Branch bronchi
Bronchiole
Right lung
Oxygen is taken into the blood from the alveoli
Air sac (alveolus)

The lower airways extract oxygen and feed it into the bloodstream

Coughs, colds and fevers

VIRUS INFECTIONS

Everyone gets virus infections of the nose and throat from time to time, and the symptoms are all too familiar:

- sneezing
- runny or blocked nose
- sore throat
- cough
- raised temperature.

There are so many different viruses which can cause these infections that it's not possible to develop lifelong immunity to them as it is to specific virus infections such as measles or mumps. We may, however, acquire some resistance to such infections as a result of being exposed to the viruses repeatedly.

As toddlers and young children start mixing more with other children – at playgroup, nursery or school – they also come into contact with a wide variety of viruses for the first time. This often means they go through a time of frequent infections which can be troublesome and worrying for you as parents. Nevertheless, it should be seen as a normal phase in which your child is coming to terms with the common viruses.

Unfortunately, because of the large number of different viruses and their changing patterns, immunisation against the common nose and throat viruses is not possible. The influenza virus, for example, is notorious for its ability to change its composition slightly so that immunity to last year's version doesn't mean you're immune to this year's. However, immunisation against 'flu is possible, provided that a vaccine against the prevalent virus is made each autumn. The jab has to be given every year, but it is not currently recommended for children unless they are known to suffer from:

- long-standing chest problems (such as asthma or cystic fibrosis)
- long-standing heart disease
- chronic kidney failure
- diabetes
- lack of immunity because of disease or medical treatment.

Don't be confused by the fact that your child may have had or been offered Hib (or *Haemophilus influenzae* type b) vaccine. This is designed to protect against the *Haemophilus influenzae* bacterium (as its name suggests), which is quite different from the influenza virus and causes quite different diseases.

UPPER RESPIRATORY TRACT INFECTIONS

These are known in doctors' shorthand as URTIs or, by some, usually younger doctors, as 'urties'. An infected child will have the symptoms of a cold, feel feverish and off colour and may refuse to eat. Occasionally, a child (especially a very young one) may develop particular feeding or breathing difficulties and need to go into hospital for observation and nursing. Usually, though, they can be looked after at home and will get better in a few days. Just make your child as comfortable as you can – in or out of bed as they like – and make sure they drink plenty of fluid. Two to three pints a day is about right for a toddler. Don't let them get too hot

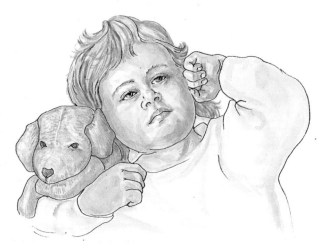

A child with a virus infection doesn't have to go to bed, but needs plenty to drink

and, if necessary, give them a medicine such as children's paracetamol to bring their temperature down.

Antibiotics

These aren't usually necessary because they don't work against viruses. After examining your child, the doctor will decide whether they are needed. Normally, they will only be prescribed for bacterial infections such as ear infections (otitis media), tonsillitis or pneumonia. There is good evidence that antibiotics may cause side effects such as a rash or diarrhoea. What's more, using them frequently and unnecessarily may encourage the growth of resistant bacteria which means that antibiotics may not work when they are really needed. And of course, it's wasting money that the NHS could otherwise use to better effect.

CASE HISTORY

Six-year-old Joel was brought to the hospital because he had been off colour for three or four days. He seemed to have had a cold and a fever and had complained of headache, and he had vomited frequently. That morning there had been some blood in the vomit.

Joel looked mildly ill, a few lymph glands could be felt in his neck, and his throat and ear drums were reddish looking. Because of the headache and vomiting it was important to rule out meningitis and a lumbar puncture was done. The spinal fluid was normal, proving that he did not have meningitis. A diagnosis of viral upper respiratory tract infection was made and he recovered without treatment.

(Both headache and vomiting may be symptoms of viral upper respiratory tract infection. Frequent vomiting may cause a small tear in the lining of the stomach resulting in blood being brought up.)

MEASLES

This is a very highly infectious disease which, once introduced into a home, will infect about 70 per cent of people who have not had it before or not been immunised against it. In a school it will infect about 30 or 40 per cent of non-immune contacts. Measles is spread by direct contact with someone who has it or through the air by coughs and sneezes.

A child with measles is infectious to others from just before the first symptoms appear to four days after the rash comes out. The time from being in contact with the disease to developing the first symptoms (the incubation period) is about 10 days.

- The first symptoms are like a cold, with a cough, fever and red eyes.

- The typical red spots appear two or three days later, first behind the ears, then spreading to the face and then all over.
- A tell-tale sign of measles which doctors look for is the appearance of Koplik's spots. These are small white spots, often said to be like grains of salt, on the insides of the cheeks, level with the back teeth.

Within a day or so of the rash coming out the child's temperature usually settles and he or she begins to feel much better. They are usually back at school in a week.

About one child in 15 with measles suffers some kind of complication such as croup (see page 30), ear infection, chest infec-tion, convulsions or, very rarely, encephalitis (swelling or inflam-mation of the brain). This last, serious, complication affects about one child in 5,000 with measles.

Immunisation against measles is now combined with mumps and rubella (German measles) immunis-ation in the MMR vaccine and is very successful. Measles epidemics used to occur every other year before immunisation was intro-duced.

The number of cases began dropping from a peak of between 600,000 and 800,000 in epidemic years when the measles vaccine was introduced in 1970 and, since MMR immunisation was started in 1988, the number of cases has declined almost to zero.

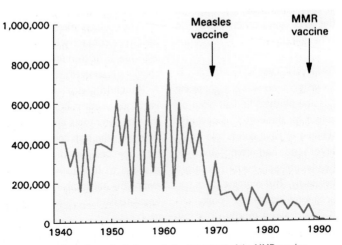

Occurrences of measles before and after the advent of the MMR vaccine.
(From *Immunisation against Infectious Disease*, HMSO, 1992)

FEBRILE CONVULSIONS

Febrile convulsions occur in about one child in 30 between the ages of six months and five years. For some reason not fully understood children's brains between these ages are prone to excess electrical activity at times of fever, and excess electrical activity in the brain often means fits (or convulsions – the words mean the same thing; sometimes, especially in America, they are called seizures). Anything that causes a fever may start off a febrile convulsion but, more often than not, it's a viral upper respiratory tract infection.

If your child has a fever:

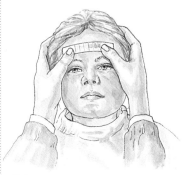

Children's paracetamol will help to bring down a raised temperature

- do not overheat him or her by putting on too many layers of clothes or overheating the room
- give a medicine such as children's paracetamol or ibuprofen to help bring the temperature down
- make sure they get plenty to drink.

Febrile convulsions look awful. When you first see one you might even think – as many parents do – that your child has died, but try and remember that they are not nearly as serious as they look. It is almost unknown for a child to come to any harm during a febrile convulsion. It may be that a very long convulsion (over 30 minutes) could harm the brain but even that is uncertain and if it does happen it is very rare. Most convulsions, in any case, stop long before that.

If your child has a febrile convulsion simply lie him or her down on the side and wait for it to stop. If it doesn't stop within 10 minutes call for a doctor or take the child to hospital. (You would be justified in dialling 999 for an ambulance at this stage if necessary.) In any case ask your doctor to see the child as soon as possible after the convulsion is over. After one febrile convulsion there is about a one in three chance of having another over the next year or so but your child will eventually outgrow this tendency. The risk gets rapidly less after the age of three, and very few children with febrile convulsions later go on to develop epilepsy. If your child has had a febrile convulsion you may be given an injection (diazepam, stesolid) to inject into his back passage to cut short any future episodes.

CASE HISTORY
Three-year-old Daniel suddenly developed a high temperature, probably as a result of a viral infection. Four hours later he seemed to faint, his whole body became stiff and then his arms and legs started to shake, his eyes rolled up and he was frothing at the mouth. This lasted for four or five minutes and then he was very sleepy. His mother took him to hospital but by the time they got there he was much better although he still had a temperature. His throat was red but otherwise he was all right. The doctors diagnosed a febrile convulsion brought on by an upper respiratory tract infection.

MENINGITIS
This is perhaps the most serious disease that doctors are on the lookout for in young children who have a fever; it is so serious because it may be rapidly fatal if not treated quickly. There are two kinds of meningitis, viral and bacterial. Viral meningitis is not serious and gets better of its own accord. Bacterial meningitis, however, needs urgent antibiotic treatment. Call the doctor immediately or dial 999 if your child:

- seems unduly ill or sleepy
- complains of severe headache
- vomits repeatedly
- develops a rash consisting of purple/blue/red spots
- complains of a stiff neck or has difficulty bending her head forward to drop her chin on to her chest.

Remember that almost all children have viral upper respiratory tract infections from time to time and few get meningitis. But if you are in doubt, play safe. A child with bacterial meningitis needs treatment very urgently.

COUGHS – VIRUSES, WHOOPING COUGH AND ASTHMA
Coughs can usually be put down to one of three main causes:

1 a viral upper respiratory tract infection – normally only lasting a few days
2 whooping cough – a serious and potentially lethal bacterial infection
3 asthma – when the cough is persistent and normally worse at night.

We will look at each of these in turn.

Viral URTI
Most coughs are the result of a viral upper respiratory tract infection

(URTI) and don't usually last long. However, if – as often happens – your child gets one infection after another, the cough will probably come back as well.

An alternative explanation is that the child may have an allergy (see page 37). In either case, a discharge from the nose is a normal symptom, although this is common in children and may occasionally have some other cause. When your child lies on his or her back, the discharge will tend to run back into the throat, causing irritation and a cough. This is often called 'the postnasal drip'.

Children in hospital are not often given cough medicines because they are not usually very effective, and some used in the past were found to upset some children. Most colds caused by a virus infection will be short-lived and all you need to do is to try to keep the child comfortable, and provide plenty to drink. A child who has a cough that persists should see a doctor so that a diagnosis can be made and appropriate treatment given. In some children coughing seems to become a habit.

Whooping cough (or pertussis)

This is especially likely to affect young children and is caused by the bacterium *Bordetella pertussis*. It starts as a cold with a cough that gets worse, with coughing spasms which last for a minute or so and make it difficult for the child to breathe. Sometimes there is the characteristic whooping sound which gives the illness its name, and the child is often sick after a bout of coughing.

The whoop is a high-pitched noise made in the child's throat when he or she breathes in after a coughing spell – cough, cough,

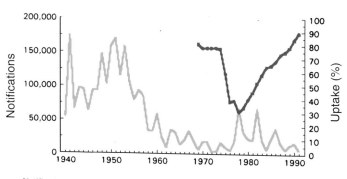

Notification (━━━) and uptake (━━━) on immunisation for whooping cough in England and Wales 1940–1991 (from HMSO)

cough . . . whoop. It varies from one child to another, and may not be very noticeable in some children, especially if they're older. Whooping cough is very distressing, and the cough may last for several weeks. It is most dangerous in young babies and it is largely to protect them that immunisation is so vital.

Only if a high percentage of the population is immunised will there be very few cases in the community, so that young babies will be protected from it before they are old enough to be immunised themselves.

● **Immunisation.** The whooping cough vaccine is effective and safe. Some years ago, there was a lot of publicity given to the possibility that it might give rise to brain damage in some children. In fact this complication is very rare indeed and some leading child specialists still dispute that it happens at all. The best evidence at present available indicates that brain damage may occur at a rate of one in every 300,000 injections (or one in every 100,000 children receiving the full course of three injections). This amounts to a very small risk. It means, for example, that the average GP immunising every baby in his or her practice would see this complication about once every 1,000 years! It's also important to

balance any such risk from the vaccine against the risk from the disease itself: whooping cough is considerably more likely to result in brain damage than the vaccine.

Until recently, babies were not given whooping cough vaccine in this country if, for example, they had an allergy or had epilepsy in their families. Today, however, there are only two real reasons for avoiding it:

● if the child is ill, immunisation should be postponed until he or she has recovered
● if the child has a severe local or general reaction to a previous dose, the next immunisation should be with diphtheria and tetanus vaccine only, rather than with the usual triple vaccine which includes pertussis.

If you have any worries about having your child immunised, talk them over with your doctor.

● **Treatment**. If your child is sick after a bout of coughing, give him or her small drinks and meals afterwards – this will help to ensure that he or she keeps some nourishment down. Sadly, there are few magic potions available to reduce the severity or duration of a bout of whooping cough! Your GP may prescribe antibiotics, especially one called erythromycin, to make the cough less severe and make the patient less infectious to others. Unfortunately, such medication must be taken early to do any good, and whooping cough is difficult to diagnose in its early stages. A baby who is severely affected may be admitted to hospital so he or she can be given oxygen quickly if necessary and treatment to prevent dehydration.

Remember that the best treatment is prevention.

CASE HISTORY

Eight-week-old baby Abigail seemed to have a cold with a runny nose and a mild cough. After four days the bouts of coughing became worse and she began to whoop and become blue in the face with her cough. She was not keeping her feeds down and was admitted to hospital.

Tests showed the high blood lymphocyte count characteristic of whooping cough but the bacterium, *Bordetella pertussis*, was not grown from her throat. She was treated with erythromycin but stayed in hospital for four days because of a persisting troublesome cough. Ten days later she was still coughing and not feeding well and she spent another four days in hospital before finally recovering.

Comment: this baby had typical whooping cough. The throat culture

may be negative if an antibiotic has been given before coming into hospital. Very young babies depend for their protection on high levels of immunisation in the community.

Asthma

Some children who have a persistent cough which is especially troublesome at night later develop asthma. In fact, this is the most common diagnosis among children attending hospital outpatient clinics because of this particular symptom.

Episodes of wheezing are characteristic of asthma: the noise comes when the child breathes out and is caused by narrowing of the air tubes, the bronchi and bronchioles. In children, the disease is almost always caused by an allergy. Usually, the child and/or other members of the family have other forms of allergy as well – such as eczema or hay fever. Asthma itself is extremely common – estimates suggest that at least 10 per cent of all children have it at some time.

The disease has actually become more widespread over the last two or three decades for reasons that are not entirely clear. Increased pollution from motor vehicles may be partly to blame but it does not seem to be the whole answer.

Most children have only mild asthma, and modern treatment with bronchodilator drugs (which open up the bronchi by relaxing the muscle in the lining) enables them to lead normal, full lives. If the child suffers frequent attacks, preventive treatment with either sodium cromoglycate (Intal) or an inhaled steroid drug may be needed. Most – although not all – children outgrow their asthma in late childhood. For further information about asthma, see our book *Understanding Asthma* in the same series.

CATARRH

The term is used to describe a clear, mucous discharge which comes usually from the nose and, as we've seen, it's very common in young children. There are two main causes:

- frequent virus infections
- an allergy called chronic allergic rhinitis which mainly affects the lining of the nose.

If your child has catarrh continuously over a long period, allergy is the most likely explanation, especially if he or she (or other family members) has some other allergic condition such as eczema or asthma. This particular kind of allergy is known as atopy, and the diseases that result as atopic diseases. Children with chronic rhinitis often develop the habit of rubbing their noses with the front of their fist or hand – the so-called 'allergic salute'.

Allergy and catarrh

Often it is not clear what's causing an allergy, or it may be many different things. One common trigger is a tiny mite called the house dust mite which is found in bedding and other soft furnishings. If your child is affected, you may be advised to try and limit his or her contact with the mites by damp dusting regularly and vacuuming his or her mattress, but it's not certain what effect this has on symptoms.

An allergy affecting the nose which comes on when the pollen count is high is called hay fever (see the book *Understanding Hay Fever* in this series). Catarrh may interfere

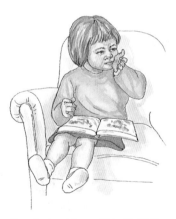

The allergic salute – a child with rhinitis will often rub her nose with the front of her hand

with drainage of your child's middle ear, causing a tendency to suffer infections of that part of the ear (otitis media, see page 42). Usually, children with catarrh improve greatly once they've been at school for a while.

SINUS PROBLEMS

The paranasal sinuses are air-filled cavities within the skull bones which drain through small holes into the cavity of the nose. They're situated within the cheek bones and the bones of the forehead.

Sinusitis

Although children don't often have symptoms caused by acute sinusitis, all viral upper respiratory tract infections involving the nose probably also affect the sinuses to some extent. When acute sinusitis does cause problems, symptoms will probably include:

- fever
- feeling generally off colour
- tenderness over the affected sinus.

You should take your child to the doctor, who will be able to prescribe an antibiotic if necessary.

● **Chronic sinusitis:** this is often a form of allergy, and the child is also likely to have other symptoms, including:

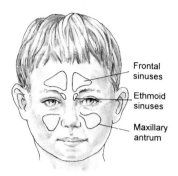

Frontal sinuses
Ethmoid sinuses
Maxillary antrum

Sinusitis can be caused by a viral infection or be a form of allergy

- a persistent cough
- a blocked or runny nose
- foul-smelling breath.

Children don't often need to have an operation to drain affected sinuses.

CYSTIC FIBROSIS

This is a serious inherited condition which affects about one in 2,000 white children. Children of other races are less likely to have it. The way in which it is inherited is called recessive; this means that both parents are well but carry the gene. Each of their children has a one in four chance of inheriting the gene from both of them and thus of being born with the condition. It affects the chest, causing a chronic cough, and the pancreas, which means that they can't digest fat and tend not to put on weight well.

Older children and adults may have nasal polyps. People with cystic fibrosis now live much longer than was the case 20 or 30 years ago, and the recent discovery of the cystic fibrosis gene has given a spur to more research and hope of an eventual cure.

KEY POINTS

✓ Children usually have more colds and coughs when they start at playgroup, nursery or school because they are meeting new viruses to which they have no immunity

✓ 'Flu vaccine is only recommended for children when they have specific health problems such as cystic fibrosis or heart disease

✓ Antibiotics don't work against viruses, so your doctor will only prescribe them if your child has a bacterial infection at the same time as a cold

✓ A baby or toddler may have a fit if he or she has a high temperature. These are called febrile convulsions and are not as serious as they look. They don't mean that your child has epilepsy

✓ At least 10 per cent of children today are thought to have asthma which has become more common in recent years and this is often the explanation for a persistent cough

Mouth and throat

The fact that you can actually see for yourself when your child has something wrong with his or her mouth makes you more likely to worry than if the problem were invisible.

YOUR CHILD'S TONGUE

Sometimes children develop raw-looking areas on their tongue. These areas are painless; they look like the lines on a map and because of that the condition is called geographical tongue. It is harmless and needs no treatment.

Tongue tie

Look under your own tongue in the mirror and you will see a narrow strip of tissue connecting your tongue with the floor of your mouth. This is called the lingual frenum and when it is very short and restricts movement of the tongue we call that tongue tie. (A small child's frenum is attached to the tongue very much nearer the tip

than yours is.) Like many parents, you may be worried about this, but in fact most children with tongue tie don't require any treatment. It does not cause a speech problem or interfere with feeding and usually, as the tongue grows, the frenum becomes attached further and

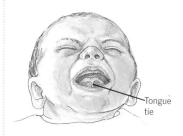

Tongue tie

Most children with tongue tie don't need treatment

further back in the mouth. This allows the front of the tongue to be moved and stuck out normally. A few children who can't stick their tongue out when they're toddlers are better off having a minor operation to cut the frenum and free the tongue. Being able to stick your tongue out is an important part of being a child!

Thrush

Lots of young babies get thrush. They develop white spots on the palate, tongue and inside the cheeks. Milk curds left in the mouth after a feed can look like thrush but, unlike thrush which sticks to the inside of the mouth, they can be easily brushed off with the tip of a spoon.

Thrush may pass downwards through the baby's bowels and infect the skin of the nappy area causing nappy rash. Most nappy rashes, however, are not caused by thrush. Some babies are infected with thrush during birth because their mother has the fungus organism responsible – *Monilia* or

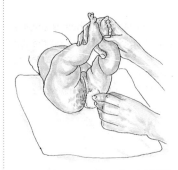

Nappy rash can sometimes be caused by thrush

Candida species – in her vagina. If so, she may need treatment, which is relatively simple.

As so often, prevention is better than cure. The best precaution against thrush is to be absolutely scrupulous about sterilising your baby's bottles and teats. Do ask your doctor or health visitor for advice if there seems to be a problem.

HERPES STOMATITIS

Herpes simplex virus infection of the mouth (herpes stomatitis) is very uncomfortable for a child – usually a toddler – who gets it. He or she will usually be feverish and develop many small painful ulcers on the lips and inside the mouth. The symptoms normally disappear after a few days; meanwhile, encourage your child to drink fluids and to eat light sloppy foods because swallowing will be painful. A new drug called acyclovir may cut the illness short.

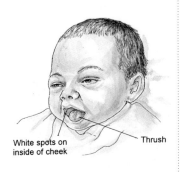

White spots on inside of cheek — Thrush

A baby with thrush has white spots inside her mouth and on her tongue

Later in life the herpes simplex virus causes cold sores on the lips and the infection can be passed to children by an adult who has one.

Children with eczema may get a serious skin infection with herpes simplex virus so if they get stomatitis or develop small blisters on the skin they should see a doctor. This is especially important if the child has been in contact with an adult with cold sores or another child with stomatitis.

SWALLOWING PROBLEMS

These don't normally last long and are the result of infections such as tonsillitis or stomatitis. Premature babies born more than four weeks early usually have difficulty swallowing because their nervous system control has not quite fully developed. They may need to be fed through a tube until they grow old enough to feed normally. Some children with cerebral palsy have problems feeding because of a lack of nervous system control of movements of the tongue and throat muscles.

SPEAKING DIFFICULTIES

Normally when we speak, the soft palate seals off the nasopharynx and stops air coming down the nose. When this doesn't happen, the person is said to be speaking nasally (talking down their nose). Obviously, when an individual has a cleft palate (see page 50) this air seal cannot be effective.

Sometimes the cleft palate may not be obvious; the palate may be too short or there may be a small cleft hidden under the covering of the palate (called a submucous cleft of the palate). This type of problem is best diagnosed by an ear, nose and throat surgeon.

DRIBBLING

All young children dribble saliva, some more than others. Sometimes it is because they have a sore throat and swallowing the saliva is painful, or, occasionally, it's the result of a more serious infection such as epiglottitis (see page 31).

Most children grow out of the habit by the time they're four, although some go on doing it regularly after that age. This is more common in children with cerebral palsy or slow development. It is often messy and socially embarrassing to the child, in which case treatment with a medication called hyoscine can help. This is often given in the form of a patch which is applied to the skin.

Sometimes mouth and tongue exercises can help and these are often supervised by a children's speech therapist. When the problem is severe and troublesome, the child's doctor may consider operating on the salivary glands or the ducts which carry the saliva from the glands into the mouth, but this is rarely necessary.

CHEMICAL BURNS

If your child should accidentally swallow something – such as a strong acid or caustic soda – which burns the mouth and throat, don't try giving him or her anything to drink as an 'antidote'. Take the child to the nearest hospital straightaway. The doctors will probably want to look into the oesophagus through a special tube (oesophagoscopy) to assess how much (or how little) damage has been done.

THROAT INJURY

A serious injury which could usually be avoided is what doctors sometimes call 'pencil injury'. What most often happens is that a child falls over with a pencil or something similar in his or her mouth, and the pencil then hits the back of the throat. Sometimes, the main artery

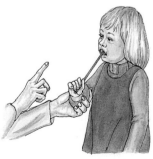

A child could hurt herself badly if she fell with a pencil or something similar in her mouth

to the brain which runs close to the back of the throat may be injured, causing a kind of stroke. This is fortunately quite rare but obviously very serious when it does happen. This is why you should do all you can to prevent it happening – never allow your child to play with a pencil or anything similar sticking out of the mouth.

KEY POINTS

✓ There's usually no need to worry if your child seems to have tongue tie as he or she will probably grow out of it without needing treatment

✓ Careful sterilisation of all your baby's bottles and teats is the best precaution against thrush infection

✓ All children dribble, but most will have stopped by the time they're four or so. Otherwise, treatment is possible for those who need it

✓ Never give milk or any other drink to a child who has accidentally swallowed something that burns the throat – just get him or her to hospital quickly

Tonsils and adenoids

Tonsils and adenoids are composed of what's called lymphoid tissue (similar to the lymph glands found throughout the body) and they form part of the body's defence against infection.

TONSILS

Look into your child's mouth and you'll easily see the tonsils – two large round masses, one on either side at the back.

In toddlers, they are usually very large and almost meet in the midline. This is perfectly normal, and the size of the tonsils is no cause for concern, provided your child is otherwise well.

In very rare cases, large tonsils and adenoids may cause problems by obstructing a child's breathing. This could be the problem if your child:

- snores
- is restless at night
- has prolonged pauses in breathing
- is sleepy in the mornings.

If you are concerned about such symptoms, ask your GP to examine your child to assess whether he or she needs to be referred to a paediatrician or an ear, nose and throat surgeon. It is important to remember, however, that most

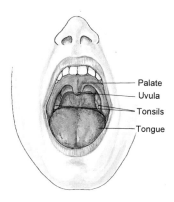

Palate
Uvula
Tonsils
Tongue

Tonsils are an important defence against infection

children with large tonsils are perfectly normal and healthy.

Sore throats

Most sore throats are simply a symptom of one of the common virus infections (see page 3). When you look into your child's mouth, the whole of the back of the mouth and throat looks red. The only treatment needed is a pain reliever such as children's paracetamol in liquid form, together with a light, soft or semi-fluid diet to make swallowing easier.

A small minority of sore throats are caused by bacteria, particularly one type called *Streptococcus*. People used to be frightened of such infections in the past because some varieties of *Streptococcus* gave rise to scarlet fever and others could be followed by rheumatic fever or inflammation of the kidneys (nephritis).

Over the last 40 or 50 years, however, there seems to have been a natural change in these diseases. Scarlet fever is now very rare in Britain and, when it does occur, it is a much milder disease than that which used to cause serious illness in children in the 1930s and 1940s. Rheumatic fever is also a rarity these days, to the extent that doctors who qualified in this country in the last 30 years have probably never seen a case. Nephritis does still occur, but not

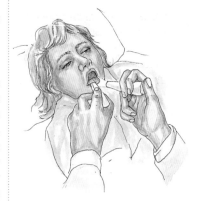

A throat examination will help the doctor assess whether your child's tonsils are normal

very often and is rarely the result of streptococcal infection.

The risk of a child with a sore throat developing any of these diseases in Britain in the 1990s is extremely small, and antibiotics are not needed as a matter of course. However, if tests do identify *Streptococcus* as the cause of an infection, a course of penicillin will rapidly clear it.

Diphtheria

Nowadays, this illness is rare in Britain, but there are still a few cases affecting unimmunised children and children from abroad. It produces a sore throat with a characteristic grey film over the tonsils and throat, and may affect the heart and nerves. It can be a very serious disease. However, a child who has a grey film over his or her throat is today much more likely to have some other infection – such as glandular fever – rather than diphtheria.

As the condition is now so rare in this country, there is no natural immunity to it. This means it is vital that children should be immunised against it in case they should come into contact with a case from abroad or travel to other parts of the world where it still occurs regularly.

Tonsillitis

In most sore throats, the whole throat is inflamed, but in tonsillitis the infection is centred on the tonsils. Your child is likely to:

- have a severe sore throat
- find it difficult to swallow
- be feverish
- look and feel unwell.

You'll see that his or her tonsils are reddened and have small beads of white/yellow pus on them. Some of the spots may run together to form a sheet. A white or grey film over the tonsils used to be seen in people with diphtheria, but today, thanks to immunisation, this is another disease which has almost disappeared.

Nowadays, a film or membrane over the tonsils is more likely to be caused by glandular fever.

Each area of the body has its own system of lymph glands to help defend against infection. The

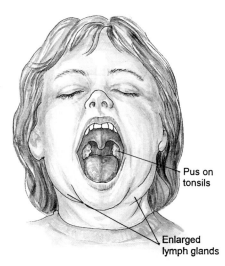

Pus on tonsils

Enlarged lymph glands

A child with tonsillitis will have a very sore throat and feel unwell

ones that protect the body from infection spreading from the tonsils are found just below the angle of the jaw. They are often enlarged in a child with tonsillitis.

Although a virus infection can cause tonsillitis, a bacterial infection is a more likely culprit than with a simple sore throat, so most doctors will prescribe a course of antibiotics to cut the attack short. Occasionally, a pocket of pus may form in the throat alongside one tonsil. This is called a quinsy, although you may also hear it referred to as a peritonsillar abscess. It is very uncommon in children, affecting adults more often, and is treated with antibiotics, together with drainage of the pus and later with removal of the tonsils.

CASE HISTORY

Two-year-old Gemma had had a cold and a cough for four days. She had been feverish and off her food. Her face was flushed and both tonsils were covered in spots of whitish pus, and she found it difficult to swallow. Her GP prescribed an antibiotic because of the tonsillitis. Her temperature settled within a few hours and by the next day she was well again.

Tonsil removal – the pros and cons

Removal of tonsils and adenoids is one of the most frequently performed of all operations. Many doctors believe that too many such operations were done in the past. Although tonsils and adenoids are often removed at the same time, this isn't always necessary – and one may be removed without the other.

Having their tonsils out means your child won't get tonsillitis any more, but it won't stop him or her getting frequent sore throats and virus infections. This is why the operation (called tonsillectomy) is only considered if your child is having unacceptably frequent bouts of tonsillitis. In fact, because such attacks tend to occur less often as a young child gets older, and often stop altogether in time, adopting a 'wait and see' policy may mean the operation turns out not to be necessary.

Although the operation is very safe and most children get over it quickly, there is sometimes bleeding from the site of the tonsils afterwards which can be difficult to stop. All ear, nose and throat surgeons will have had experience of dealing with these difficult and worrying cases, which is why most don't want to be pressurised into doing the operation without good reason.

Very occasionally, the operation may have to be done because the child has a quinsy or truly enormous tonsils which block off the throat.

ADENOIDS

Under a microscope, the adenoids look just like the tonsils. They lie at the back of the throat just above the roof of the mouth, and you can only see them with the special medical instruments used by ear, nose and throat surgeons.

Big adenoids may block the flow of air through a child's nose, making them snore or breathe through their mouth. They may also affect the child's ears, causing inflammation or fluid accumulation in the middle ear (see page 42). This happens when large adenoids press on the tube which connects the air-filled cavity

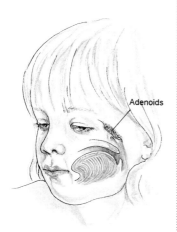

Adenoids

of the middle ear with the throat. If this tube (known as the eustachian tube) is blocked, the pressure in the middle ear falls, fluid accumulates and infection may set in. Swal-

lowing opens out the throat end of the eustachian tube and so the pressure of the air in the middle ear can become equal with that in the throat. Incidentally, this is why swallowing will usually relieve the sensation of 'popping ears' that you sometimes get when you climb or descend rapidly in an aeroplane or a car.

CASE HISTORY

Seven-year-old Jenny had had a blocked nose and snored at night for the last two years. At first the decision was taken to remove her adenoids; some months later, however, she seemed to be much better and it was decided not to proceed with the operation.

Three years later the same symptoms occurred again, although this time the ear, nose and throat surgeon felt that, as she was now nearly eleven and her adenoids could be expected to shrink of their own accord fairly soon, she did not need an operation. She was treated with nose drops and improved but, because her symptoms persisted, her adenoids were eventually removed.

Comment: it can be difficult to decide at what point surgery is necessary. Spontaneous improvement is common and a period of 'wait and see' is often a sensible policy.

Adenoid removal

An operation to remove the adenoids (adenoidectomy) is usually done either because of blockage of the air flow through the nose or middle-ear problems of the kinds described earlier and in the section on otitis media and glue ear on pages 42–44.

KEY POINTS

- ✓ Tonsils and adenoids are an important part of the body's defences against infections

- ✓ Your toddler's tonsils may look large, but this is nothing to worry about if he or she is otherwise well

- ✓ A child with tonsillitis will need antibiotics, but most sore throats are caused by a virus and just need to be soothed with children's paracetamol

- ✓ These days, surgeons prefer not to remove a child's tonsils without very good reason because there is a small but real risk of complications after the operation

Neck lumps

As a parent, you probably worry whenever your child develops a lump in his or her neck. However, this is very common and rarely serious. Nevertheless, if you are worried about any lump in your child's neck ask your GP to look at it. It's one of the most common reasons why children are taken to a doctor.

LYMPH GLANDS

The most common explanation for a neck lump is that a lymph gland has become enlarged. We all have these glands and they often increase in size in response to infection. Their function is to prevent the infection from spreading throughout the body. Many of the infections that cause the swelling are unimportant

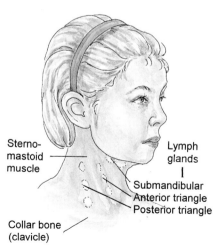

Sterno-mastoid muscle

Lymph glands

Submandibular
Anterior triangle
Posterior triangle

Collar bone (clavicle)

The three places on the neck where lymph glands swell in response to infection and cause no other symptoms. Swollen neck lymph glands are usually in one of three places. The glands which swell with tonsillitis are under the jaw (submandibular).

You may hear doctors talking about glands being in the anterior or posterior triangle. The neck, on each side, is divided by the muscle (sternomastoid muscle) which goes from the bony mastoid process behind the ear down to the inner part of the collar bone (clavicle). In front of that muscle is referred to as the anterior triangle of the neck and behind it the posterior triangle. The lymph glands in these triangles often swell with infections around the head and neck.

Most swollen glands will settle of their own accord but seek your doctor's advice if:

- the gland (or glands) is large

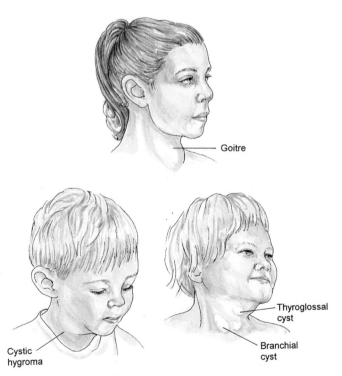

Other types of swelling on the neck which need medical attention

(more than about half to three-quarters of an inch across)

- it is tender or red
- it seems squelchy rather than firm to the touch
- it is growing
- it stays the same for longer than a few days
- you can also feel swollen glands in your child's armpits or in the groins
- your child is ill or has lost weight.

OTHER NECK SWELLINGS

Goitre

This is the name given to a swelling of the thyroid gland. It is a much broader swelling than enlarged lymph glands and straddles the front of the neck between the bottom of the larynx and the top of the breast bone. Some babies are born with a goitre but it is much more common in the early teens.

Anybody with a goitre should be seen by a doctor so that their thyroid gland can be tested.

Thyroglossal cyst

This forms a round swelling in the midline of the neck below the chin. It is attached to the tongue and therefore moves upwards when the child sticks out his or her tongue. It needs to be removed by an operation.

Branchial cyst

This may appear to one side of the neck near the sternomastoid muscle, and it too will need to be removed by surgery.

Cystic hygroma

This is an unusual and rare, but sometimes troublesome, swelling in the neck. It is a non-malignant tumour of lymph vessels. It starts any time in the first two or three years of a child's life, usually beginning in one posterior triangle. Sometimes these grow very big and spread on to the chin. It is possible to remove them by surgery, but the operation can be very difficult.

KEY POINTS

✓ A lump in the neck is one of the most common reasons why children are taken to the doctor

✓ Most lumps are swollen lymph glands which are part of the body's response to an infection

✓ If you are worried, it's worth taking your child to see your GP as there are some rarer causes of lumps which may need treatment

The larynx

The larynx is the voice box and its front part forms your Adam's apple. Inside is a pair of horizontal folds which regulate the flow of air from your lungs when you speak. These are the vocal folds or cords. Your ability to speak doesn't, of course, depend only on your vocal cords – your lips, tongue and palate are all important as well.

Above the vocal cords is a projection called the epiglottis which you can't see when looking into your throat unless it is swollen by epiglottitis (see page 31). Below the vocal cords, the larynx leads to the trachea (or windpipe) which divides inside the chest into two bronchi which carry air to the lungs.

The important symptom which

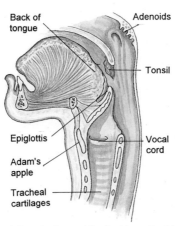

Back of tongue

Adenoids

Tonsil

Epiglottis

Vocal cord

Adam's apple

Tracheal cartilages

The larynx is the voice box, and the front forms the Adam's apple

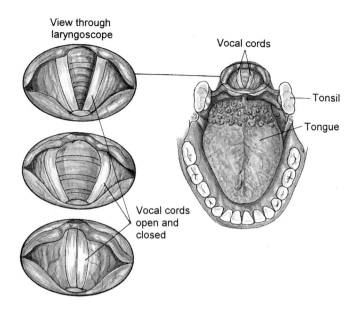

View through laryngoscope

Vocal cords

Tonsil

Tongue

Vocal cords open and closed

What the larynx looks like seen through an instrument called a laryngoscope

points to trouble in your child's larynx is called stridor.

STRIDOR – THE MAIN SYMPTOM

This is the name given to a shrill, high-pitched noise which you can hear as your child is breathing in. It is usually caused by a narrowing of some part of the larynx. (A noise heard when your child breathes out, on the other hand, is usually caused by asthma.)

Newborn babies

When your baby is born, the walls of his or her larynx may be soft and floppy so that it tends to collapse inwards when the baby breathes in – this is known variously as:

- congenital laryngeal stridor
- laryngomalacia
- floppy larynx.

Your baby will probably be well apart from the noisy breathing, and the condition will improve over the next 12 months as the larynx grows. Your baby may need to be examined by an ear, nose and throat surgeon if:

- breathing is laboured
- weight gain is slower than normal

- the stridor shows no signs of improving with time.

The child may be admitted to hospital for an examination known as laryngoscopy, which is done under general anaesthetic using an instrument called a laryngoscope.

Occasionally, a baby who has stridor from birth may have some problem other than a floppy larynx. He or she may have some abnormality in the vocal cords or the windpipe may be narrowed just below the vocal cords – a condition known as subglottic stenosis. In severe cases, the child may need an operation to widen the windpipe, but this will often be put off for a while so that the windpipe can grow. In the most serious cases, where the baby has real problems breathing, it may be necessary to overcome the obstruction. There are two possible ways of doing this, although they are only needed in exceptional cases:

- endotracheal intubation – passing a plastic tube through the baby's mouth or nose, past the point of obstruction
- tracheostomy – making an opening through the neck directly into the windpipe.

Most babies born with stridor don't run into any trouble and get over the problem in time. If, however, the stridor suddenly gets

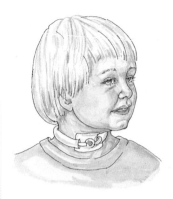

Occasionally, a tracheostomy (or opening in the windpipe) is needed to help a child to breathe

worse and the baby's breathing becomes laboured, he or she should be taken straight to hospital so that doctors can assess whether any treatment is needed.

Toddlers
When stridor comes on in a toddler or a child of school age, the reason is normally either:

- an infection in the larynx
- a foreign body in the windpipe (see page 33).

INFECTION OF THE LARYNX

Croup
Some children are prone to develop stridor while suffering from virus infections – often called croup. Usually the illness is quite mild and they get over it quickly. Measles may occasionally start with stridor,

but sometimes it seems to be allergy rather than infection that is responsible for the symptom.

When the stridor is only mild, you may be able to relieve it by sitting your child in a hot bath so that he or she is breathing moist air.

Laryngo-tracheo-bronchitis

This more severe infection is usually caused by a virus similar to the one that causes 'flu. It has this triple-barrelled name because it normally produces inflammation not only in a child's larynx (laryngitis) but also in the trachea and bronchi.

The illness generally comes on over a day or two, and the child develops fairly severe stridor with quite a loud noise and has difficulty breathing. Your child may well find the symptoms alarming and is likely to feel quite frightened. Unless the symptoms are very mild and quickly over, he or she is likely to need to go into hospital for observation. However, a calm atmosphere and some moistening of the air should bring about a complete recovery in a few days.

Unfortunately, antibiotics can't help because it is a virus infection, although sometimes inhaled adrenaline or an inhaled or injected steroid drug may be given. In rare, very severe cases, endotracheal intubation may be necessary, and this would mean the child being nursed on an intensive care unit.

EPIGLOTTITIS

Inflammation of the epiglottis is usually caused by the bacterium *Haemophilus influenzae* type b. The symptoms are similar to those of laryngo-tracheo-bronchitis but are much more severe and much more serious. They come on quickly – within a few hours – and include:

- severe stridor
- the child seems very ill
- sore throat
- difficulty swallowing.

The child may also:

- dribble
- develop a cough.

It is vital to get an expert diagnosis and treatment as soon as possible because, without it, epiglottitis can lead to complete blockage of the larynx and the child could die. Do not delay. If your child has these symptoms (as opposed to mild croup) take him to hospital as soon as possible. Dial 999 if necessary. In this situation never try to examine your child's throat yourself using a wooden blade or a spoon handle to press down the tongue, as this could cause spasm of the larynx and blockage of the airway.

Epiglottitis must always be treated in hospital. First, the doctor will examine the child with a laryngoscope, usually under a short general anaesthetic in the operating theatre or the intensive care unit. The diagnosis is confirmed when the epiglottis is seen to be red and swollen. A plastic tube is then inserted through the baby's mouth or nose so there is no longer any risk of the airway becoming obstructed. The patient can then be given antibiotics to treat the infection, but, once the airway has been protected, the danger is past and recovery should only take a few days. Occasionally, if the doctor has difficulty inserting the tube, it may be necessary to make an opening in the front of the windpipe (or trachea, which is why the procedure is called a tracheostomy).

The *Haemophilus influenzae* type b bacterium which is responsible for epiglottitis can also be one of the causes of meningitis. Fortunately, both illnesses have become much rarer since immunisation with the Hib vaccine was introduced in 1992. This is another instance where prevention is very much better than cure.

KEY POINTS

✓ A high-pitched, shrill noise when a child is breathing in – known as stridor – is a sign that there may be a larynx problem

✓ Some babies are born with stridor and most grow out of it by the time they're a year old

✓ Mild stridor in a toddler may be eased by letting your child breathe in moist air while in a hot bath

✓ Some viral infections of the larynx may mean a short stay in hospital for observation or treatment

✓ Epiglottitis is a potentially serious infection, but fortunately it can be prevented by making sure your child has the Hib immunisation

Foreign bodies in the ear, nose and throat

IN THE LARYNX

Stridor (the breathing-in noise described in the previous chapter) which comes on suddenly always makes a doctor think that the child may have inhaled a foreign body. If so, the size and nature of the object concerned will determine whether it stays in the larynx or passes down into the trachea, bronchi or lungs.

Peanuts in particular are notorious for producing severe inflammation in the lungs – which is why throwing them in the air and catching them in your mouth is extremely dangerous. Adults who show children how to do this (with peanuts or anything else) as a party trick could be putting their lives at risk.

Choking

Any time your child has a severe choking spell, you should make sure he or she is seen by the doctor afterwards, especially if you aren't sure whether he or she has coughed up all the material responsible. Any symptoms – such as a persistent cough or wheeze – after choking mean that your child should be examined by a doctor as soon as possible. The emergency procedures used when a child chokes are shown on pages 34–35.

EARS AND NOSES

Young children are prone to get foreign bodies into strange places! Small objects, such as beads, little balls of tissue paper or the rubber tyres off toy cars may find their way into virtually any body opening.

A child with something in his or her ear will find the ear painful and be unable to hear through it. A foreign body in the nose will cause a breathing blockage in one side of the nose and a persistent discharge. If your child has a persistent discharge from one nostril, especially if it's streaked with blood, you should take him or her to the doctor.

Removing such objects often needs considerable skill, and it is usually best done in an ear, nose and throat department – your GP will refer you if necessary.

Nose bleeds

The medical term for nose bleeds is epistaxis. It is common in children and usually caused by damage to blood vessels in the nose caused by small fingers. Other possible causes include infections and allergies in the nose or objects (foreign bodies) being inserted into the nose. Much more rarely it may be a sign of a blood problem causing bleeding.

If your children have nose bleeds sit them upright on a chair, with the head tilted forwards to that the blood does not run back into the throat, and press firmly (but no need to hurt!) on the soft part of the nose. In most cases the bleeding will stop fairly quickly. If it does not, the child should see a doctor so that the bleeding can be stopped, if necessary by packing the nose with a bandage.

A child who has frequent or very bad nose bleeds should also see a doctor so that any necessary tests can be done. It might be necessary to 'burn off' some of the blood vessels at the front of the nose which give rise to bleeding. Sometimes, applying an ointment regularly just inside the nostrils will help prevent bleeding.

WHEN CHOKING IS AN EMERGENCY

When children get something stuck in their larynx, it can cause a complete blockage and prevent them from breathing. Their life may be at risk unless you do something quickly to relieve the obstruction:

1 If the child is still a baby: lay him along your forearm holding his chest firmly in your hand. His head should be below his chest. Give him four light slaps on the back with your other hand

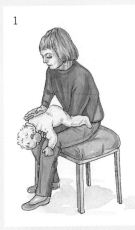

1

Emergency choking: babies

2 Turn the child upside down over your knee, with her head down towards the floor and hit

2

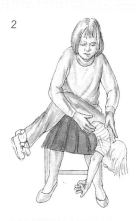

Emergency choking: child

her back between the shoulder blades several times

3 If the choking doesn't stop, you should perform Heimlich's manoeuvre. This can be done in two ways:

A

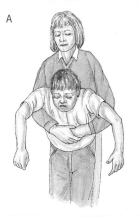

Heimlich's manoeuvre

A put your arms around the child from behind, joining your hands in front of his stomach as in a bear hug; then give a sharp pull into his stomach – the idea is to create enough sudden pressure to make the object causing the blockage pop out like a Champagne cork

B

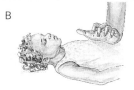

B with the child lying flat on her back press quickly with the palm of your hand into her stomach to produce the same effect

Using excessive force may cause damage, and you need to use less with a smaller child, but you simply have to do the best you can because this is an extreme emergency

Putting your fingers down a child's throat to feel for the foreign body may occasionally work if the object is relatively large. However, it can be disastrous if the object is pushed further in, so only try it as a last resort if the other methods haven't worked

✓ Never show children how to throw peanuts and catch them in their mouths. Any such small object can lodge in the lungs and cause inflammation

✓ A child who continues to wheeze or cough after a severe choking attack should be seen by a doctor to check that the lungs are clear of foreign matter

✓ Removing foreign bodies from a child's ear or nose is a job best left to the experts at the hospital

✓ Nose bleeds are common in children and are usually the result of damage to small blood vessels caused by the child's fingers. Consult your doctor if your child has frequent attacks

Allergy

When we say someone has an allergy, we mean that his or her body reacts in a particular way to food or to substances found in the environment. The problem is very common, and produces a wide variety of symptoms which can affect different parts of the body. Any substance which causes the reaction is known as an allergen. When the symptoms come on suddenly and very soon after eating or contact with the allergen, it may be possible to identify a single cause. Often, however, and especially when the problems are longstanding, there could be several possible allergens, and it isn't always possible to find a single culprit.

SUDDEN (OR ACUTE) REACTIONS

The kind of allergic reaction that comes on suddenly has had a lot of coverage in the media recently. Peanuts have featured prominently in press and TV reports, but other foods which may be troublesome include milk, fish, shellfish and eggs, although almost any food can be the cause of allergy in some people.

Symptoms of an acute allergic reaction may include:

- a blotchy red skin rash, often with weals (urticaria)
- swollen or painful joints
- wheezing
- sneezing
- swelling in the throat
- in severe cases, collapse and shock (known as anaphylaxis or anaphylactic shock); in most people, the reaction isn't severe enough to lead to collapse.

Together with your doctor, you need to try and identify the offending allergen. If it turns out to be something edible, it's often helpful to get a dietitian's advice as it isn't always obvious which foods contain it. Your doctor may suggest that you keep a non-sedative antihistamine to give your child if a reaction should start or if he or she is exposed to the antigen accidentally.

You may also be given a preloaded syringe so that you can inject adrenaline under your child's skin at the onset of a reaction. There has been a lot of debate in the medical profession about which children really need this treatment. Some experts in childhood allergy feel it should only be given to parents whose child has suffered a particularly severe episode.

LONGSTANDING PROBLEMS

Children with longstanding (or chronic) allergies usually have the type known as atopy. It may affect the lungs (asthma), the skin (eczema) or the nose (rhinitis), and these are known as atopic diseases. Often atopy may run in families, with several members having the same or different diseases. For example, you may have eczema, your child asthma and your brother or sister rhinitis. Any one person could have all three conditions, and it's common for children to have asthma and eczema at the same time. In some people, the diseases seem to alternate – as one gets worse, the other gets better.

Rhinitis

When rhinitis comes on only at certain times of the year, usually in spring and early summer in response to grass and pollens, it is called hay fever. However, some children have it all year round, when it's known as perennial rhinitis.

- **All year round:** a child with perennial rhinitis is always snuffly and has a constantly runny or blocked nose. When he or she lies down at night, the discharge from the nose may trickle back into the throat and cause a troublesome cough.

Hay fever

This is so easy to recognise that you can probably diagnose it yourself. When the pollen count rises, your child will:

- have a clear nasal discharge
- sneeze frequently
- have prickly, red, watering eyes.

- **Treatment:** most children with either kind of rhinitis will be treated with anti-allergy drugs, taken either by mouth or as nose drops. The ones most often taken by mouth are the antihistamines, and the latest types do not cause drowsiness which was the big disadvantage of older versions.

There are several kinds of nose drops used to treat allergic rhinitis. Some act quickly by shrinking the swollen lining of the nose. They can be useful to relieve nasal blockage and to allow other kinds of nose drops or sprays to get into the nose and work more effectively. However, it's not wise to use them for long periods – one or two days at a time is enough. Drops and sprays which can be used on a long-term basis to suppress inflammation and swelling of the nose linings come in two kinds: sodium cromoglycate (Rynacrom) and steroid solutions such as beclomethasone (Beconase).

KEY POINTS

✓ A sudden allergic reaction may be caused by something your child has eaten. Common culprits include peanuts, milk, eggs, fish and shellfish

✓ Allergic conditions such as asthma, eczema and rhinitis often run in families

✓ A child with a constantly running or blocked nose may have perennial rhinitis which can usually be controlled with simple treatment

The ears

HOW THEY WORK

The ear consists of:

- the external ear – the pinna and the ear canal
- the middle ear
- the inner ear

- the ear drum – a thin membrane which separates the ear canal from the middle ear.

The middle ear is an air-filled space in the bone of the skull which contains a chain of three tiny bones called the hammer (malleus), the

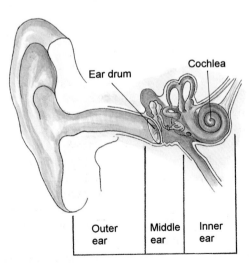

The ear consists of three parts: the inner, middle and outer ear

anvil (incus) and the stirrup (stapes). These little bones (or ossicles) transmit the sound vibrations from the ear drum to the inner ear. The space of the middle ear is connected to the throat by means of the eustachian tube and also to the air-containing spaces (called the mastoid air spaces) in the rounded part of the skull bone below the ear.

The inner ear has two parts. One, called the cochlea, is the organ of hearing. It sends messages through the nerve of the ear (the auditory nerve) to the brain where the final analysis and perception of sound take place. The other part, called the labyrinth, is concerned with maintaining our balance.

DISEASES OF THE EAR

The outer ear
● **The pinna:** this may be small or of an unusual shape, or placed unusually low down on the face nearer to the chin. These may simply be variations of normal but sometimes they may be a pointer to something else such as a kidney abnormality. The doctors looking after your newborn baby may wish to check on the baby's kidneys with an ultrasound scan if the ears look unusual.

If your child has ears which stick out (sometimes called 'bat ears') and gets a lot of teasing from other children, the problem can be

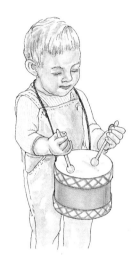

corrected by a plastic surgeon. Some babies are born with small skin tags in front of the ear. They're called accessory auricles and can be removed surgically or, if they're very small, a short length of cotton is tied tightly round them so they shrivel up and fall off in a few days.

● **The ear canal:** as the ear canal is lined with skin, it is susceptible to problems such as eczema and boils. This part of the ear can also become infected – a condition known as otitis externa.

You may notice a lot of wax in your child's ear, but it doesn't usually cause any problems and needs no treatment. It is a natural secretion whose purpose is to cleanse the ear and it normally works its way to the edge of the ear of its own accord. You don't need to

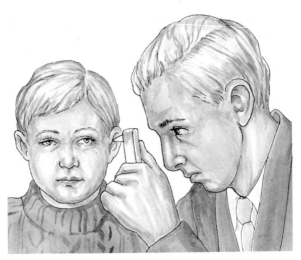

An ear examination will help the doctor diagnose otitis media

wipe out your child's ear with cotton buds and in fact this can do damage to the ear canal. By compressing the wax, it can also prevent it from escaping from the ear.

The middle ear

• **Otitis media:** this is the name given to an infection of the middle ear. Along with the nose and throat, this part of the ear is often mildly inflamed when your child has a cold or one of the common virus infections, and it can also be a complication of measles. However, severe inflammation centred on the middle ear is often the result of bacterial infection. Otitis media is common in children, especially in those under six, because the eustachian tube is relatively short so it's easy for infections to spread from the nose and throat.

A child who is old enough will tell you he or she has earache and will be feverish and generally off-colour. Younger ones may simply seem ill and feverish and may vomit, but won't be able to tell you that they have earache. Your GP can diagnose otitis media by examining your child's eardrum through an instrument called an auroscope – the eardrum will look red and bulging.

Most children get better after a few days without treatment, although you should give them a pain-relieving medicine such as children's paracetamol. Your GP will probably prescribe an antibiotic, although not everyone is convinced that it makes much difference. At one time, a small cut was made in the eardrum to relieve pressure in the middle ear, but this operation (called myringotomy) is not often done today.

When there is a discharge of pus from the ear, it means the eardrum must have ruptured, but it will usually heal up by itself quite quickly. Sometimes, however, the infection persists, which results in longstanding perforation of the eardrum. Dealing with this kind of infection, known as chronic otitis media, usually needs the expert skills of a hospital ear, nose and throat department. Once your child has got over an attack of otitis media, his or her hearing will need

checking to make sure it has returned to normal.

When a child keeps on having otitis media, it may be because of enlarged adenoids, and the problem is also common in children with a cleft palate.

• **Glue ear:** sometimes called secretory or serous otitis media, this condition is common in young children. Instead of being filled with air, the middle-ear cavity contains clear, sticky fluid and this prevents the child from hearing properly. Treatment is designed to restore the hearing to normal, but in fact hearing can come and go regardless.

Decongestant medicines and nose drops are given to reduce any swelling in the lining of the child's nose and throat and to keep the eustachian tube open so fluid can drain from the middle-ear cavity and be replaced by air. Alternatively, a surgeon may try to drain the middle ear by making a small incision in the eardrum (myringotomy) and inserting a small plastic tube called a grommet through the drum to allow the fluid to escape. The grommets usually drop out on their own after a few months, allowing the eardrum to heal. The ear, nose and throat surgeon may also want to consider whether removing your child's adenoids would be helpful.

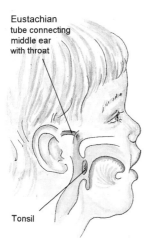

Eustachian tube connecting middle ear with throat

Tonsil

Otitis media is common in children under six years because of the shortness of the eustachian tube

The number of operations performed for glue ear has seen a big increase in recent years, and some surgeons feel that too many have been done. Glue ear often gets better without treatment anyway, which means it's important to be as sure as possible that the operation is really necessary. It is done under a general anaesthetic and, although modern anaesthesia is very safe, it should never be given unnecessarily.

There is also concern that some children may end up with permanent scarring of the eardrum after grommets have been inserted. This is why it's wise to avoid rushing into surgery too soon, but there's no doubt that many children have benefited from it. Persistent hearing loss causing speech development to be delayed, frequent inattention or problems at school are reasons for considering surgery if medical treatment hasn't helped. As with all medical decisions, it's a matter of balancing the pros and cons. On the one hand, no one wants to do unnecessary operations and, on the other, everyone wants the operation to be offered to those children with a serious, persisting hearing loss who could benefit from it.

You may be advised that your child shouldn't swim with grommets in, but generally doctors say it's OK provided he or she wears ear plugs and a bathing cap. Diving and jumping in are banned, however, as there's a risk of water getting into the middle ear via the eustachian tubes.

CASE HISTORY

Five-year-old James was noticed by both his parents and his teacher to have had an occasional hearing problem over the last two years. He was referred by his school doctor to an ear, nose and throat surgeon who found signs of fluid in the middle ear on both sides; in addition the ear drum did not move well on carrying out a test called tympanometry, although his hearing seemed satisfactory. As a result of this history of variable hearing difficulty and the finding of 'glue ear' the surgeon decided to remove the boy's tonsils and adenoids and to insert grommets into the ear drums.

After the operation James was well and his hearing was normal, although a year later the grommet on the left had come out and his hearing on that side deteriorated slightly. Another grommet was inserted and after that he had no more trouble.

Comment: grommets often fall out from their position in the drum. They may not need to be replaced unless the child's hearing deteriorates.

- **Mastoiditis:** in the days before antibiotics, infection in the middle-ear cavity often spread to the mastoid air spaces in the bone of the skull just behind the ears. The rounded prominences of bone you can feel just behind each ear are called the mastoid processes, and they will be tender and painful if your child has acute mastoiditis. Until antibiotics began to be used to treat otitis media, operations to drain pus from the bone were common, but nowadays they're rarely needed.

The inner ear

Problems in this part of the ear are less common than those affecting the middle ear. When hearing loss originates in the inner ear, it's called nerve deafness, while the kind that originates in the middle ear is known as conductive deafness. Some babies are born deaf as a result of abnormalities of the inner ear. Some are born with nerve deafness because their mothers caught German measles (rubella) during pregnancy, but now that most women are immunised against rubella with the MMR vaccine before conception, this problem has become rare. Very occasionally, a child's nerve of hearing may be affected by disease such as meningitis or a tumour, and some drugs can cause damage to the nerve. Mostly these are special antibiotics used only in hospital, and doctors try to avoid the problem by checking carefully on the blood levels of these drugs whenever they are used to make sure they stay within safe limits.

Labyrinthitis is a virus infection – rare in children – which strikes the inner ear and affects balance. It usually comes on fairly suddenly, causing fever, dizziness and vomiting, but sufferers normally recover in a few days.

Benign paroxysmal vertigo is an uncommon condition which affects toddlers. It seems to be due to a problem in the organ of balance in the inner ear, but no one knows what causes it. The child may suddenly feel dizzy and wobbly on his or her feet and may feel frightened and run to the mother for

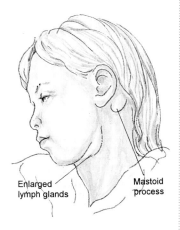

Enlarged
lymph glands

Mastoid
process

Occasionally, infection may spread from the middle ear to the mastoid processes

comfort. In this situation, you may notice that the child's eyes have developed jerky movements from side to side – doctors call this nystagmus. As the symptoms occur for short periods of a few minutes at a time, doctors sometimes mistakenly diagnose some kind of fit or epilepsy. However, epilepsy treatment does not seem to help, and the problem goes by itself after a few weeks or months.

KEY POINTS

- ✓ Don't use cotton buds or anything else to clean inside your child's ears. It isn't necessary and can cause damage

- ✓ A child who's had persistent middle-ear infections, especially glue ear, should have a hearing test to make sure it hasn't been affected

- ✓ Doctors will consider carefully whether a child needs to have grommets inserted in his or her ears to drain off fluid as the operation has risks as well as benefits

- ✓ Dizziness may be a symptom of inner-ear infection, but this is relatively uncommon and doesn't usually need any treatment

Hearing and speech development

Your baby will start to react by smiling when you speak to him or her at around six to eight weeks, and to coo and gurgle shortly after that. By three or four months, he or she will turn the head to look for the source of a sound at the same level as the ear – turning to sounds above or below the ear comes slightly later. Double syllables – da-da, ba-ba – start to appear at about eight months and by the time the babies are a year old, they'll be saying two or three proper words. Remember that there's a difference between da-da which is purely a baby noise and learning to say dada to mean father. During the second year, your child will gradually learn more single words and at around two years old start putting them together into simple sentences. Of course, he'll only learn to speak if he's spoken to, so it's important that you talk to him all the time. If you're concerned about his speech development, have him checked over at your local baby clinic.

HEARING TESTS

In some countries, newborn babies have their hearing checked routinely, but this is not yet the case in Britain. Experts disagree about testing methods, and even in countries where testing is carried out, the best tests may not be used. Old approaches which rely on observing a baby's bodily response to sound are being replaced by more objective tests:

- AER (or brain-stem auditory evoked response) measures the electrical activity at the base of the brain caused by sound reaching the ear.
- OAE (or transient evoked otoacoustic emission) relies on the discovery that the

inner ear itself actually produces sound while it is processing sounds reaching the ear. Although it is too soft to be heard, this sound can be detected by a sensitive microphone placed in the outer ear – proving that the inner ear is working. It's still new and not generally available as yet, but it's quick and easy to do, and may become the best way of routinely testing the hearing of very young children.

It is essential to spot nerve deafness as early as possible in a child's life so that steps can be taken to keep the degree of handicap to a minimum.

ROUTINE CHECKS

All babies need to have their hearing tested, and this is normally done by your health visitor at the clinic at around six or seven months. For this check, she'll probably use a special high-tone rattle and make high-pitched (psss) and low-pitched (ooo) sounds with her own voice. More complex methods are used for older children, using either the voice or a sound-

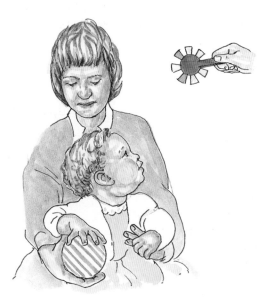

The health visitor uses a special rattle to test your baby's hearing

producing machine (audiometer). A child whose hearing loss needs further assessment may be referred to an ear, nose and throat surgeon who can provide special tests, including:

- tympanometry – assessing the movement of the ear drum when varying pressures are applied to it
- electrical tests such as AER – see page 47.

Remember that if you're worried about your child's hearing or speech at any time, you should ask for her to be checked over. Most health districts now have child development centres or children's care and assessment units, often attached to the district hospital paediatric department. These can offer a more detailed assessment of a child's development, including speech and hearing, when necessary.

Some very intelligent children who can hear perfectly don't speak until they're three or four (Einstein was a late speaker!), but it's important to have a full assessment of a child whose speech development is slow. That way, if there is a problem, any necessary action to deal with it can be started as soon as possible. You can't just assume that it's just because your child is destined to be a genius like Einstein! Even a baby as young as six months can wear a hearing aid if he or she needs one.

KEY POINTS

✓ Children only learn to speak if they're spoken to, so talk to your baby as much as you can

✓ Your health visitor will probably check your child's hearing at around six or seven months, but you should ask for a check any time if you're worried

✓ Some perfectly healthy children don't talk till around the age of four, but slow developers should be checked just in case

✓ Children as young as six months can wear a hearing aid

Your newborn baby

THE MOUTH

There is no need to worry if your new baby has a line of small white spots on either side of the midline of the palate. These are called epithelial pearls and they are normal – thrush would not line itself up neatly like that.

Yours may be one of the small number of babies who are

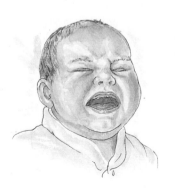

When a baby is born with a tooth, it will have to be removed

born with a tooth. However, these teeth aren't normal, and need to be removed to stop them coming loose and finding their way into the baby's chest.

CLEFT LIP AND PALATE

Babies born with cleft lip and/or palate may be distressing to look at at first, but modern surgery can improve their appearance enormously. Most newborn baby units now have a collection of 'before and after' pictures to show to parents so that they can see what can be done.

The operation on a baby's lip is usually done at about three or four months of age and the palate is operated on later – usually between six and 15 months.

Later the child will need to be checked for possible ear problems such as glue ear and may need orthodontic treatment. Speech

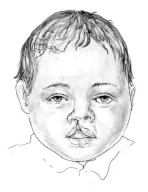

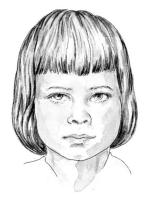

Before operation
for cleft lip

2 years after

An operation to repair a cleft lip is usually done at around three to four months

therapy may also be necessary for some children.

BLOCKED NOSES

Babies can't breathe through their mouths very well, so they have difficulty if they can't breathe through their noses. The problem is usually caused by catarrh and swelling of the lining of the nose because of a virus infection or an allergy. A brief course of nose drops may help but if your baby is very young, they may not be used as the problem may become worse when the drops are stopped.

Very rarely babies may be born with the back of the nose closed off by bone. This is called choanal atresia. If both sides of the nose are affected the baby will need an operation quite soon, but if the blockage only affects one side surgery may be postponed, often for several years.

Stridor – or noisy breathing – in newborn babies is covered on pages 29–30.

KEY POINTS

✓ Some children may need speech and language therapy following surgery for hare lip or cleft palate

✓ Young babies can't breathe easily through their mouths; a child with a blocked nose should be seen by a doctor

Preventing problems

Although you can't prevent all of the problems described in previous pages, some you can. The three main approaches to prevention are immunisation, not smoking and early hearing tests – and we'll look at each in turn.

IMMUNISATION

This is vitally important. Whooping cough (pertussis), measles, mumps,

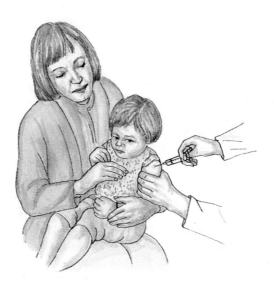

Immunisation can now protect children from many common illnesses, some of which used to kill

YOUR CHILD'S IMMUNISATIONS

Vaccine		Age	Comments
Diphtheria/tetanus/ pertussis (D/T/P), polio and Hib	(1st dose) (2nd dose) (3rd dose)	2 months 3 months 4 months	Primary course
Measles/mumps/ rubella (MMR)		12–18 months	Can be given at any age over 12 months
Booster D/T and polio, MMR (if not had previously)		4–5 years	
BCG		10–14 years	
Booster tetanus and polio		15–18 years	

From *Immunisation against Infectious Disease*, HMSO, 1992

rubella, diphtheria and *Haemophilus influenzae* type b (Hib) may all cause serious problems in a child's throat and ears, and there are effective vaccines against all of them.

Immunisation checklist
- By six months: three doses of diphtheria/tetanus/pertussis (D/T/P), Hib and polio
- By 15 months: measles/mumps/ rubella (MMR)
- When school starts: fourth diphtheria and tetanus, and polio; MMR if missed earlier
- Between 10 and 14 years: BCG
- Before leaving school: fifth polio and tetanus

SMOKING
This is a major cause of ear and throat problems. Passive smoking in children is a background factor in many diseases. If you smoke, your children are almost twice as likely to have respiratory problems, including asthma. and are 30 per cent more likely to have glue ear compared with the children of non-

smokers. Quite apart from the effect this has on the health of the children themselves, it has been estimated that parental smoking increases the amount the NHS spends on them by nearly £150 million each year.

EARLY HEARING TESTS

Keeping appointments for hearing checks means that a child who is born with nerve deafness will be identified as early as possible and steps can then be taken to limit the resulting handicap.

And finally...

As we've seen, disorders affecting a child's nose and throat are extremely common – especially while he or she is very young. When your child seems to have one such ailment after another, you may worry that he or she is more often ill than well and will turn up for that first job interview still suffering from otitis media! Don't despair. You may find it hard to accept at the moment, but the fact is that most of the problems discussed in this booklet are simply a normal if difficult part of growing up and will disappear naturally in time.

Useful addresses

CHILD ISSUES IN GENERAL

Action for Sick Children
Argyle House
29–31 Euston Road
London NW1 2SD
Tel: 0171 833 2041
Web site:
www.inclusive.co.uk/support/sickch.htm

Formerly known as the National Association for the Welfare of Children in Hospital (NAWCH), the association promotes the welfare of sick children in hospital and at home. There is a national network of branches and services including a Parents Advice Line, a wide range of publications including a quarterly magazine, and a centralised library covering the emotional welfare of sick children. Help and support for parents are offered through local branches.

Royal College of Paediatrics and Child Health
50 Hallam Street
London W1N 6DE
Tel: 0171 307 5600

The BPA is the main professional organisation for British paediatricians. Enquiries on child health matters are referred to appropriate experts and written information sheets for parents on various topics are available.

The National Children's Bureau
8 Wakeley Street
London EC1V 7QE
Tel: 0171 843 6000
Web site: www.ncb.org.uk

The Bureau collects and disseminates information about children and promotes good practice in children's services through research, policy and practice development, membership, publications, conferences, training and an extensive library and information service.

ALLERGY

Action Against Allergy
PO Box 278
Twickenham
Middlesex TW1 4QQ
Tel: 0181 892 2711
Web site: www.thesite.org.uk/5163

This organisation offers information and support for allergy sufferers and publishes a newsletter. A large list of books and pamphlets is available on request. It also raises funds for allergy research.

British Allergy Foundation (BAF)
Deepdene House
30 Bellegrove Road
Welling
Kent DA16 3PY
Tel: 0181 303 8525
Allergy Helpline: 0891 516500

The BAF also offers information and support and raises funds for research.

The National Society for Research into Allergies
PO Box 45
Hinckley
Leicestershire LE10 1JY
Tel: 01455 851546

The society offers practical advice,

diet sheets and introductions to local members. It publishes several booklets and a quarterly magazine, holds an annual symposium and contributes to research.

ASTHMA

National Asthma Campaign (NAC)
Providence House, Providence Place
London N1 0NT
Tel: 0171 226 2260
Asthma Helpline: 0345 010203
(Monday to Friday 9 a.m. – 7 p.m.)
Web site: www.asthma.org.uk

The NAC provides support and information, and funding for research into asthma. There is a wide range of education material, a Junior Asthma Club (ages six to 11), and a quarterly magazine. Children's activity holidays are arranged in association with the National Eczema Society.

CLEFT LIP AND/OR PALATE

Cleft Lip and Palate Association (CLAPA)
138 Buckingham Palace Road
London SW1 9SA
Tel: 0171 824 8110
Email: clapa@mcmail.com
Web site: www.clapa@mcmail.com

CLAPA offers support for parents through a network of groups and aims to support research. There is an annual newsletter and booklets are available. There is a specialist service for parents and health professionals experiencing difficulties feeding newborn babies with cleft palate.

CYSTIC FIBROSIS

Cystic Fibrosis Trust
11 London Road
Bromley
Kent BR1 1BY
Tel: 0181 464 7211

The Trust offers advice and support to families and supports research and care of patients with cystic fibrosis. There are branches throughout the UK. Holiday caravans may be rented at nominal charge by families of cystic fibrosis patients.

CYSTIC HYGROMA

Cystic Hygroma Support Group
Villa Fontana
Church Road
Worth
Crawley
West Sussex RH10 7RS
Tel: 01293 885901

This is a small contact group. There is a periodic newsletter and an annual meeting at the organiser's home (Mrs Pearl Fowler). The group provides information and contact with other parents.

DEAFNESS

The National Deaf Children's Society
15 Dupperin Street
London EC1Y 8PD
Helpline: 0171 250 0123 (Mon–Fri, 10 a.m.– 5 p.m.)
email: ndcs@ndcs.org.uk

The society offers support, information and advice. There are local group meetings. The society's magazine *TALK* is published quarterly.

Breakthrough Deaf/Hearing Integration
Alan Gaila House
The Close
Westhill Campus
Bristol Road
Selly Oak
Birmingham B29 6LN
Tel: 0121 472 6447

Breakthrough offers information, support, contacts and advice. There is a varied programme of activities including workshops and courses.

Index